The Heart Of A Midwife: Daily Devotionals for Christian Midwives

Delightful Devotionals

CONTENTS

Introduction

Day 1: The Miracle of Birth

Day 2: Guiding Light in Labor

Day 3: Strength in Labor

Day 4: Embracing New Beginnings

Day 5: Comforting the Fearful

Day 6: The Sacred Bond of Motherhood

Day 7: Celebrating Diversity in Birth

Day 8: Nurturing Holistic Well-being

Day 9: Trusting the Divine Timing

Day 10: The Gift of New Life

Day 11: Empowering Women in Birth

Day 12: Finding Peace in the Delivery Room

Day 13: Joy in the Midst of Pain

Day 14: Wisdom in Birthing Choices

Day 15: Honoring the Sacred Journey

Day 16: Compassion in the Delivery Room

Day 17: Surrendering to the Miracle

Day 18: Grace in Birthing Challenges

Day 19: The Role of Prayer in Birth

Day 20: A Midwife's Calling

Day 21: Gratitude for the Gift of Life

Conclusion

Notes

Introduction

Welcome to "The Heart Of A Midwife: Devotionals for Midwives." This unique collection of daily reflections is crafted to inspire and uplift those devoted to the noble profession of midwifery. As midwives, you stand at the intersection of science and the miraculous, guiding new life into the world with skill, compassion, and reverence. This devotional is designed to accompany you on this sacred journey, providing moments of spiritual reflection and inspiration amidst the demanding yet profoundly rewarding nature of your work.

In the tapestry of childbirth, each day unfolds a new chapter, and within these pages, you'll find moments of respite, wisdom, and connection with God. Whether you are a seasoned midwife or embarking on this fulfilling path, This book invites you to pause, reflect, and draw strength from the spiritual dimensions of your calling. Each day offers a verse, reflection, journal questions, and prayer, providing a holistic approach to nurturing your spiritual well-being as you, in turn, nurture new life.

May this devotional journey deepen your connection with the sacred art of midwifery, reminding you of the profound impact you have on the lives you touch. May it be a source of strength, inspiration, and encouragement as you continue to play a vital role in the beautiful narrative of birth.

Day 1: The Miracle of Birth

Verse of the Day:

Psalm 139:13-14 (NIV) - "For you created my inmost being; you knit me together in my mother's womb. I praise you because I am fearfully and wonderfully made; your works are wonderful, I know that full well."

Reflection:

Today, we embark on a journey into the awe-inspiring miracle of birth, guided by the profound words of Psalm 139. This scripture beautifully acknowledges the intricate craftsmanship involved in the creation of every life. As a midwife, you step into a sacred space, witnessing the miracle of God's design unfolding in the womb. The divine act of knitting together life serves as a reminder of the intimate connection between the Creator and the created.

In embracing the role of bringing new life into the world, reflect on the profound responsibility entrusted to you. Each birth is a testament to the intricate plan and purpose woven by God. It's an acknowledgment that, as a midwife, you play a pivotal role in the symphony of creation. This reflection invites you to stand in awe of the Creator's wisdom and express gratitude for the privilege of participating in the miracle of birth.

As you embark on this devotional journey, let Psalm 139 guide you in recognizing the sacredness of your calling. Find joy in knowing that each birth is a testimony to the wonders of God's creation, and your role is an integral part of this divine masterpiece.

Journal:

1. How does the acknowledgment of being fearfully and wonderfully made influence your perspective on the miracle of birth?

2. Reflect on a specific moment in your midwifery journey where you felt the presence of God's craftsmanship in the birthing process.

3. In what ways can you express gratitude for the privilege of participating in the divine masterpiece of birth?

Prayer:

Heavenly Father, as I embark on this devotional journey, I am in awe of the miracle of birth that you have entrusted to me as a midwife. May your presence be felt in every birthing room, and may my hands be guided by your wisdom. I express gratitude for the privilege of participating in the sacred act of bringing new life into the world. Amen.

Day 2: Guiding Light in Labor

Verse of the Day:

Psalm 32:8 (NIV) - "I will instruct you and teach you in the way you should go; I will counsel you with my loving eye on you."

Reflection:

In the profound journey of childbirth, where emotions and physicality intertwine, the midwife assumes a pivotal role as a guide and source of strength. Psalm 32:8 delicately emphasizes the divine promise of instruction and counsel. It's a reassurance that, even in the intricate and sometimes unpredictable dance of labor, there is a source of wisdom beyond the physical realm.

As you reflect on this verse, consider the sacred space you inhabit during the birthing process. Your role as a guiding light involves not only the application of medical knowledge but also a spiritual attunement to the needs of both the mother and the newborn.

In the quiet moments of labor, acknowledge the profound impact of seeking and trusting in God's guidance. Let this reflection deepen your understanding of the divine connection between your work and the unfolding miracle of life.

Journal:

1. In what ways have you experienced God's guidance in the labor process as a midwife?

2. How does the assurance of being instructed and counseled by God influence your approach to supporting mothers in labor?

3. Reflect on a specific instance where you felt a divine presence guiding you during a challenging labor.

Prayer:

Gracious God, in the sacred moments of labor, I seek your guidance and wisdom. Instruct me, teach me, and counsel me with your loving eye on both the laboring mother and myself. May your divine presence be felt in every step of the birthing journey. Amen.

Day 3: Strength in Labor

Verse of the Day:

Philippians 4:13 (NIV) - "I can do all this through him who gives me strength."

Reflection:

Today, reflect on the profound truth embedded in Philippians 4:13, acknowledging that your strength in the challenges of labor is sourced from God.

As a midwife, you often witness the incredible strength of mothers in the birthing process. Consider the ways in which drawing upon the strength given by God empowers both you and the mothers you serve.

Take a moment to contemplate the spiritual resilience that underlies the physical and emotional demands of childbirth.

Journal:

1. How have you experienced the strength provided by God in challenging moments during labor?

2. In what ways can acknowledging God as the source of strength impact your approach to supporting mothers through difficult aspects of childbirth?

3. Reflect on a specific instance where you witnessed a mother drawing strength from her faith during labor.

Prayer:

Almighty God, I recognize that my strength and the strength of the mothers I serve come from You. Grant us the resilience and courage needed in the challenges of labor. May Your strength be evident in every birthing room. Amen.

Day 4: Embracing New Beginnings

Verse of the Day:

Lamentations 3:22-23 (NIV) - "Because of the Lord's great love we are not consumed, for his compassions never fail. They are new every morning; great is your faithfulness."

Reflection:

Today, meditate on the profound truth in Lamentations 3:22-23, acknowledging the grace and faithfulness of God in the birthing process.

As a midwife, you play a significant role in welcoming new life into the world. Reflect on the compassion and love inherent in this miraculous process. Consider the ways in which each birth is a testament to God's unfailing faithfulness and the opportunity for new beginnings.

Embrace the sacred nature of your work as you witness the arrival of each precious life.

Journal:

1. How do you see God's great love and faithfulness in the new beginnings of each birth?

2. Reflect on a particular birth experience that reminded you of the compassion and grace of God.

3. In what ways can you bring an awareness of God's faithfulness into your daily interactions with expectant mothers?

Prayer:

Heavenly Father, I am grateful for the opportunity to witness and participate in the miracle of new beginnings. May Your love and faithfulness be evident in every birth, filling each moment with grace and compassion. Amen.

Day 5: Comforting the Fearful

Verse of the Day:

Isaiah 41:10 (NIV) - "So do not fear, for I am with you; do not be dismayed, for I am your God. I will strengthen you and help you; I will uphold you with my righteous right hand."

Reflection:

Today, reflect on the powerful words of Isaiah 41:10 and consider the significant role you play as a midwife in providing comfort and reassurance.

The birthing process can be accompanied by fear and uncertainty, and your presence brings a sense of God's comforting embrace. Contemplate how you can embody the promise of God's presence and strength during these moments.

Recognize the impact of your compassionate care in alleviating fear and fostering a sense of security for expectant mothers.

Journal:

1. How have you witnessed the comforting presence of God in the birthing experiences you've been a part of?

2. In what ways do you provide reassurance and support to mothers who may be feeling fearful during labor?

3. Reflect on a specific instance where you felt God's strength upholding you in your role as a midwife.

Prayer:

Gracious God, thank You for being a source of comfort and strength. As a midwife, help me embody Your reassuring presence, bringing peace to those in moments of fear. Uphold me with Your righteous right hand as I fulfill this sacred role. Amen.

Day 6: The Sacred Bond of Motherhood

Verse of the Day:

Titus 2:4 (NIV) - "then they can urge the younger women to love their husbands and children."

Reflection:

Today, meditate on the significance of nurturing the sacred bond between mothers and their newborns, as highlighted in Titus 2:4.

As a midwife, you witness the early moments of this profound connection. Consider the role you play in fostering love, care, and support during this critical period.

Reflect on the impact your guidance can have on the foundation of a mother's relationship with her child. Recognize the beauty of your contribution to the building blocks of family bonds.

Journal:

1. How do you actively support and encourage mothers in building a strong bond with their newborns?

2. Reflect on a memorable experience where you observed the profound connection between a mother and her child during the birthing process.

3. In what ways can you continue to nurture and promote the sacred bond of motherhood in your role as a midwife?

Prayer:

Gracious Father, thank You for the gift of motherhood and the sacred bonds that form during childbirth. Guide me as a midwife to support and nurture these connections, fostering love and warmth in the early moments of family life. Amen.

Day 7: Celebrating Diversity in Birth

Verse of the Day:

Galatians 3:28 (NIV) - "There is neither Jew nor Gentile, neither slave nor free, nor is there male and female, for you are all one in Christ Jesus."

Reflection:

Today's reflection centers on the beautiful diversity present in the birthing experience, inspired by Galatians 3:28. As a midwife, you encounter people from various backgrounds, each with a unique story.

Consider the significance of being part of a process that unifies people, transcending cultural, social, and gender differences.

Embrace the diversity in the birthing room as a reflection of the unity found in Christ. Recognize the privilege you have in contributing to the shared experience of bringing new life into the world.

Journal:

1. How do you celebrate and honor the diverse backgrounds and stories of the families you assist in childbirth?

2. Reflect on an experience where you witnessed the beauty of unity amidst diversity during a birthing process.

3. In what ways can you continue to create an inclusive and supportive environment for families from various walks of life?

Prayer:

Heavenly Father, thank You for the richness of diversity You bring into the world. Help me appreciate and celebrate the unique stories and backgrounds of the families I assist in childbirth. May Your love and unity be evident in every birthing experience. Amen.

Day 8: Nurturing Holistic Well-being

Verse of the Day:

1 Thessalonians 5:23 (NIV) - "May God himself, the God of peace, sanctify you through and through. May your whole spirit, soul, and body be kept blameless at the coming of our Lord Jesus Christ."

Reflection:

Today's reflection draws inspiration from 1 Thessalonians 5:23, emphasizing the holistic approach to caring for the well-being of mothers.

As a midwife, you play a crucial role in ensuring not only the physical health of mothers but also addressing the spiritual and emotional aspects.

Reflect on the significance of nurturing the whole being during the birthing process. Consider how you integrate a holistic approach in your care, recognizing the interconnectedness of spirit, soul, and body. Your commitment to the comprehensive well-being of mothers contributes to a more profound and meaningful birthing experience.

Journal:

1. In your role as a midwife, how do you address the spiritual and emotional well-being of the mothers you assist?

2. Reflect on a specific instance where you witnessed the positive impact of a holistic approach in the birthing process.

3. How can you continue to enhance your practice to ensure the comprehensive well-being of mothers under your care?

Prayer:

Gracious God, thank You for the reminder that our well-being involves the spirit, soul, and body. Grant me wisdom and compassion to care for mothers holistically, contributing to their overall health and well-being. Amen.

Day 9: Trusting the Divine Timing

Verse of the day:

Ecclesiastes 3:1 (NIV) - "There is a time for everything, and a season for every activity under the heavens."

Reflection:

Today's reflection centers around Ecclesiastes 3:1, inviting you to embrace the divine timing of the birthing process. As a midwife, you navigate the intricacies of timing during childbirth, recognizing that each moment is part of a greater purpose.

Reflect on how you trust in the divine order of the birthing journey. Consider the significance of being present and patient, acknowledging that there is a time for every stage and activity under the heavens.

Your role involves not just technical expertise but also a deep understanding of the natural rhythms and timing that God has ordained in the miracle of birth.

Journal:

1. How do you approach and navigate the different stages of the birthing process, considering Ecclesiastes 3:1?

2. Reflect on a moment where the divine timing of a birth left a lasting impact on you.

3. In what ways can you communicate the concept of divine timing to the mothers you assist, fostering a sense of trust and peace?

Prayer:

Heavenly Father, thank You for the reminder that there is a time for everything under the heavens. Grant me patience, wisdom, and discernment as I navigate the divine timing of the birthing process. May Your presence bring comfort and assurance to both mothers and midwives. Amen.

Day 10: The Gift of New Life

Verse of the Day:

James 1:17 (NIV) - "Every good and perfect gift is from above, coming down from the Father of the heavenly lights, who does not change like shifting shadows."

Reflection:

In the realm of midwifery, each birth is a testament to the miraculous and divine. James 1:17 beautifully encapsulates the essence of bringing new life into the world.

It serves as a poignant reminder that every infant cradled in the arms of its mother is a gift, a manifestation of the unchanging love and grace bestowed from the heavenly lights. Take a moment to reflect on the profound responsibility and privilege embedded in ushering these little miracles into existence.

As a midwife, you are intricately connected to the divine narrative of life's continuation. In your hands rests the ability to witness and nurture the journey of a new life. Embrace this gift with gratitude, acknowledging the sacred trust bestowed upon you. Let the verse be a source of inspiration, reminding you that your role extends beyond the clinical to the spiritual, as you participate in the profound dance of creation.

Journal:

1. How does the verse resonate with your experiences in witnessing new life?

2. In what ways do you view your role as a midwife as a conduit for divine gifts?

3. Take a moment to journal about a memorable birth that affirmed the preciousness of new life.

Prayer:

Heavenly Father, thank you for the incredible gift of life. As I continue to serve in the sacred space of childbirth, grant me wisdom and compassion. Help me recognize the divine nature of each new life and guide my hands in nurturing and protecting these precious gifts. Amen.

Day 11: Empowering Women in Birth

Verse of the Day:

Proverbs 31:25 (NIV) - "She is clothed with strength and dignity; she can laugh at the days to come."

Reflection:

In the journey of birth, Proverbs 31:25 beautifully captures the essence of strength and dignity that envelops a woman.

As a midwife, reflect on your empowering role in supporting and uplifting women during childbirth. Consider the profound impact you have in fostering an environment where women can face the uncertainties of labor with strength and dignity.

Proverbs 31:25 invites you to celebrate the resilience and courage within every woman you assist, recognizing that through your care, they can approach the days to come with laughter and confidence.

Journal:

1. How do you see Proverbs 31:25 reflected in the women you've assisted during childbirth?

2. Share a memorable experience where you witnessed the strength and dignity of a mother during labor.

3. As a midwife, how can you continue to empower and uplift women in the birthing process?

Prayer:

Heavenly Father, I thank You for the strength and dignity You clothe women with, as beautifully expressed in Proverbs 31:25. Grant me the wisdom and compassion to empower and uplift the women under my care during childbirth. May they find confidence and laughter in the days to come. Amen.

Day 12: Finding Peace in the Delivery Room

Verse of the Day:

John 14:27 (NIV) - "Peace I leave with you; my peace I give you. I do not give to you as the world gives. Do not let your hearts be troubled and do not be afraid."

Reflection:

The delivery room can be a space filled with a mix of anticipation and apprehension. John 14:27 reminds us of the peace that transcends worldly understanding.

As a midwife, reflect on your role in creating a peaceful and calming atmosphere during childbirth. Consider how your presence and care can bring a sense of tranquility, helping both mothers and families navigate the intensity of the delivery room.

John 14:27 invites you to be a bearer of the peace that comes from a higher source, offering comfort and assurance in moments of uncertainty.

Journal:

1. How do you currently contribute to creating a peaceful environment in the delivery room?

2. Share a moment when you witnessed the impact of a calm and peaceful atmosphere during childbirth.

3. In what ways can you enhance your role in providing peace and reassurance to mothers and families?

Prayer:

Gracious God, thank You for the peace You generously give, as spoken of in John 14:27. As I serve in the delivery room, may Your peace flow through me, bringing comfort and calmness to all present. Help me be an instrument of Your peace. Amen.

Day 13: Joy in the Midst of Pain

Verse of the Day:

Psalm 30:5 (NIV) - "For his anger lasts only a moment, but his favor lasts a lifetime; weeping may stay for the night, but rejoicing comes in the morning."

Reflection:

The journey of labor often brings both physical and emotional challenges. Psalm 30:5 reminds us of the transient nature of difficulties and the promise of joy that follows.

As a midwife, reflect on the role you play in supporting women through the painful moments of labor, helping them find strength, hope, and even joy. Consider the resilience and courage displayed by mothers in the face of hardship.

Psalm 30:5 invites you to acknowledge the dawn of rejoicing that follows the night of weeping, recognizing the beauty in bringing life.

Journal

1. How do you witness moments of joy and hope during labor despite the challenges?

2. Share an experience where you saw the resilience of a mother bringing forth joy after a challenging labor.

3. In what ways can you enhance the support you provide to bring moments of rejoicing to women in labor?

Prayer:

Gracious Father, thank You for the promise of joy that follows moments of weeping, as mentioned in Psalm 30:5. Grant me the wisdom and compassion to guide and support women in labor, helping them find strength, hope, and joy. Amen.

Day 14: Wisdom in Birthing Choices

Verse of the Day:

Proverbs 2:6 (NIV) - "For the Lord gives wisdom; from his mouth come knowledge and understanding."

Reflection:

In the process of childbirth, choices abound, each carrying significance for both mother and child. Proverbs 2:6 directs our attention to the divine source of wisdom.

As a midwife, reflect on the importance of seeking God's wisdom in making birthing choices. Consider how divine knowledge and understanding can guide you in supporting mothers through decisions that impact their birthing experience.

Proverbs 2:6 encourages a reliance on God's wisdom, recognizing that the choices made in the delivery room are part of a broader tapestry of God's plan for each life.

Journal:

1. How do you incorporate divine wisdom into the birthing choices you encounter?

2. Share an experience where seeking God's wisdom led to positive outcomes in a birthing situation?

3. In what ways can you encourage mothers to seek God's guidance in their birthing choices?

Prayer:

Heavenly Father, I acknowledge Your wisdom as the ultimate guide in the birthing process. Grant me discernment and understanding as I navigate birthing choices, ensuring alignment with Your divine plan. Amen.

Day 15: Honoring the Sacred Journey

Verse of the Day:

Psalm 104:14 (NIV) - "He makes grass grow for the cattle, and plants for people to cultivate—bringing forth food from the earth."

Reflection:

In the intricate design of life, Psalm 104:14 reminds us of God's provision and the cyclical nature of creation. As a midwife, reflect on the profound journey into motherhood that unfolds with each birth.

Consider the sacredness of this experience, akin to the nurturing provision described in the verse. Recognize that your role is intertwined with the divine rhythm of life, cultivating an environment where new beginnings are nurtured.

Psalm 104:14 invites you to honor and cherish the sacred journey each mother embarks upon, acknowledging the beauty and significance of bringing new life into the world.

Journal:

1. How does your role as a midwife contribute to honoring the sacred journey of motherhood?

2. Reflect on a particular birthing experience where you sensed the sacredness of the journey.

3. In what ways can you incorporate a sense of reverence and awe into your daily practice?

Prayer:

Gracious God, I thank You for the sacred journey of motherhood. May Your presence be felt in every birthing room, and may I honor the beauty of new life as part of Your divine creation. Amen.

Day 16: Compassion in the Delivery Room

Verse of the Day:

Colossians 3:12 (NIV) - "Therefore, as God's chosen people, holy and dearly loved, clothe yourselves with compassion, kindness, humility, gentleness, and patience."

Reflection:

Colossians 3:12 serves as a poignant reminder of the virtues to embrace, especially in the delivery room. As a midwife, reflect on the significance of providing compassionate care to both mothers and newborns.

This verse invites you to clothe yourself in qualities that mirror God's love and embody the sacred nature of childbirth.

Consider the impact of approaching each delivery with compassion, kindness, humility, gentleness, and patience. In doing so, you become a vessel through which God's love and care are expressed, creating a supportive and nurturing environment for the miracle of birth.

Journal:

1. How can you intentionally incorporate compassion into your interactions during childbirth?

2. Reflect on a moment where your compassionate care made a meaningful difference for a mother.

3. In what ways does embodying the virtues mentioned in Colossians 3:12 enhance the birthing experience for both mothers and newborns?

Prayer:

Gracious Father, I seek Your guidance in embodying the virtues of compassion, kindness, humility, gentleness, and patience in my role as a midwife. May Your love shine through my actions, bringing comfort and peace to those I serve. Amen.

Day 17: Surrendering to the Miracle

Verse of the Day:

Jeremiah 29:11 (NIV) - "For I know the plans I have for you, plans to prosper you and not to harm you, plans to give you hope and a future."

Reflection:

Embrace the profound truth in Jeremiah 29:11 as you contemplate the miraculous nature of childbirth. Surrender to the divine plans unfolding in the delivery room.

Reflect on the significance of being part of a process designed by God, where each birth holds a unique purpose and promise. Consider how surrendering to God's plans can bring hope, reassurance, and a sense of purpose to both you as a midwife and to the mothers you assist.

Jeremiah's words remind you that the miracle of birth is woven into a broader tapestry of divine intentionality.

Journal:

1. How does surrendering to God's plans influence your approach to each birth?

2. Reflect on a moment where you witnessed the unfolding of a miraculous plan during childbirth.

3. In what ways can you convey the message of hope and a future to expectant mothers under your care?

Prayer:

Heavenly Father, I surrender to Your plans for each miraculous birth. Grant me wisdom and discernment as I navigate the sacred journey of childbirth, bringing hope and assurance to those in my care. Amen.

Day 18: Grace in Birthing Challenges

Verse of the Day:

2 Corinthians 12:9 (NIV) - "But he said to me, 'My grace is sufficient for you, for my power is made perfect in weakness.' Therefore, I will boast all the more gladly about my weaknesses, so that Christ's power may rest on me."

Reflection:

Reflect on the grace that transcends the challenges encountered in the birthing process. Consider the profound truth that, in moments of weakness, divine power is perfected.

As a midwife, acknowledge the vulnerabilities inherent in childbirth and find solace in the sufficiency of God's grace. This verse invites you to embrace challenges with a spirit of gratitude, recognizing that Christ's power is most evident in moments where human strength falters.

Think about how God's grace empowers you to navigate difficulties and support mothers through every birthing challenge.

Journal:

1. How have you experienced the sufficiency of God's grace in challenging birthing situations?

2. Reflect on a specific instance where you witnessed divine power manifesting in a moment of weakness.

3. In what ways can you extend the concept of grace to the mothers you assist, fostering a sense of strength amid challenges?

Prayer:

Heavenly Father, thank you for the abundant grace that sustains me in the midst of birthing challenges. May Your power be made perfect in my moments of weakness, and may I, in turn, be a vessel of Your grace to those I serve. Amen.

Day 19: The Role of Prayer in Birth

Verse of the Day:

Philippians 4:6 (NIV) - "Do not be anxious about anything, but in every situation, by prayer and petition, with thanksgiving, present your requests to God."

Reflection:

Explore the profound impact of prayer on the birthing journey. Reflect on the invitation to exchange anxiety for a spirit of prayerful surrender. As a midwife, acknowledge the significance of offering prayers and petitions during the birthing process.

Meditate on the transformative nature of these moments, recognizing the divine comfort and guidance that prayer brings.

Consider how integrating prayer into the birthing experience contributes to a sense of peace and trust in God's providence.

Journal:

1. How have you observed the role of prayer positively influencing the birthing experience for mothers?

2. Reflect on a specific instance where prayer played a significant role in navigating a challenging moment during childbirth.

3. In what ways can you encourage and facilitate prayerful moments for mothers in your care?

Prayer:

Gracious God, thank you for the gift of prayer that brings peace and comfort in the birthing room. May my prayers be a source of strength and assurance for the mothers I assist, allowing them to experience Your divine presence. Amen.

Day 20: A Midwife's Calling

Verse of the Day:

Isaiah 6:8 (NIV) - "Then I heard the voice of the Lord saying, 'Whom shall I send? And who will go for us?' And I said, 'Here am I. Send me!'"

Reflection:

Delve into the profound calling embedded in the heart of midwifery. Reflect on Isaiah's response to God's call and consider your own willingness to answer the call to serve in the realm of childbirth.

Think about the unique privilege and responsibility that comes with being a midwife, recognizing it as a divine calling.

Explore how your service aligns with God's invitation to bring forth new life into the world and contribute to the well-being of mothers and newborns.

Journal:

1. What aspects of midwifery do you consider as part of your divine calling?

2. How has your understanding of your role as a midwife evolved over your career?

3. In what ways do you sense God's guidance and presence in the midst of your calling as a midwife?

Prayer:

Gracious Lord, thank you for the calling to serve as a midwife. May I embrace this divine calling with humility, compassion, and a deep sense of purpose. Guide me in every birth, and may Your presence be felt in the sacred moments of new beginnings. Amen.

Day 21: Gratitude for the Gift of Life

Verse of the Day:

Psalm 127:3 (NIV) - "Children are a heritage from the Lord, offspring a reward from him."

Reflection:

In the final day of this devotional journey, reflect on the profound gratitude inspired by the gift of life.

Contemplate the significance of being a vessel through which new life is brought into the world. Recognize the sacred responsibility and immense joy that comes with assisting in the birth process.

Cultivate a heart full of gratitude for the privilege of participating in the miracle of life as a midwife.

Journal:

1. How does your work as a midwife contribute to your sense of gratitude for life?

2. Can you recall a specific moment in your career that deepened your appreciation for the gift of life?

3. In what ways can you express gratitude for the privilege of being a midwife?

Prayer:

Heavenly Father, I thank you for the gift of life and the opportunity to serve as a midwife. May my heart be filled with gratitude for the privilege of participating in the miracle of birth. Grant me the wisdom and compassion needed to continue this sacred work. Amen.

Conclusion

As we conclude this devotional journey, we recognize the depth of your dedication and the sacred nature of your work. Each day has been a glimpse into the spiritual dimensions of midwifery, a profession that intertwines the miraculous with the everyday. As a midwife, you embody a unique blend of scientific expertise and compassionate care, bringing new life into the world with grace and skill.

Through these reflections, we've explored the significance of your role in guiding mothers through the sacred journey of childbirth. Your commitment to the well-being of both mothers and newborns is truly admirable, reflecting the very essence of a calling. The verses, reflections, questions, and prayers shared here were crafted to provide moments of solace, inspiration, and connection with the divine, acknowledging the spiritual depth inherent in your profession.

As you carry the memories of these sacred moments forward, may they serve as a reservoir of strength, wisdom, and spiritual fortitude. May you continue to find joy in the miracles you witness, strength in the challenges you face, and fulfillment in the profound impact you have on the lives you touch.

In every birth you attend, in every life you bring into the world, remember that you are part of something extraordinary. Your dedication, compassion, and skill make a difference, leaving an indelible mark on the beautiful tapestry of human existence.

May your journey as a midwife be continually blessed, and may you always find sacred moments in the service of bringing new life into the world.

With warmest wishes and gratitude,

Delightful Devotionals